HERBAL REMEDIES FOR PNEUMONIA

Harnessing And Unlocking Herbal Wisdom For Targeting Respiratory Wellness, Effective Recovery And Healthy Living

DR. CARDEN KYRIE

DISCLAIMER

The only goal of this book is informational. Every effort has been taken by the author and publisher to ensure that the information provided is accurate. But the material in this book is given "as is," without any express or implied representation, warranty, or condition as to its accuracy, completeness, or suitability for any particular purpose.

Any loss, damage, or injury resulting from using the information in this book, or from any action or decision made as a result of such use, will not be covered by the author's or publisher's liability. It is recommended that readers seek the assistance of a certified specialist for guidance specific to their situation.

The opinions and viewpoints conveyed in this book belong to the author and may not necessarily represent the official stance or policies of any specified organizations or people. Any likeness to real-life occurrences, places, or people—living or deceased—is wholly coincidental.

No specific product, service, or therapy discussed in this book is endorsed by the author or publisher. Any reference to goods or services is made only for informative reasons and is not intended as a recommendation or endorsement.

Before making any judgments or acting on any information, readers are urged to independently confirm it all. Any unfavorable effects or repercussions arising from the usage of the material included in this book are disclaimed by the author and publisher.

By using this book, you consent to absolving the publisher and author of any and all claims, obligations, or losses resulting from your use of the material in it.

I appreciate your cooperation and understanding.

TABLE OF CONTENTS

CHAPTER ONE

INTRODUCTION TO PNEUMONIA

THE VALUE OF HERBAL TREATMENTS FOR CHEST PAIN

Because they may be useful in controlling and reducing the symptoms of this respiratory illness, herbal treatments for pneumonia are receiving more and more attention. The common and potentially dangerous respiratory infection known as pneumonia is characterized by inflammation of one or both lungs' air sacs. It frequently stems from bacteria, viruses, or fungi and can produce a variety of respiratory system-related symptoms. The use of herbal remedies and other complementary and alternative ways to manage pneumonia is becoming more popular due to the problems caused by antibiotic resistance and adverse effects from traditional therapies.

The potential of herbal therapies to provide a more all-encompassing and natural approach to treatment makes them significant in the context of pneumonia. The anti-inflammatory, antibacterial, and immune-boosting qualities of many herbal medicines are well known, and they can help the body fight off the infection. Furthermore, compared to pharmaceutical interventions, herbal remedies frequently have fewer side effects, making them a potentially safer option, particularly for people who may be sensitive to or intolerant of conventional pharmaceuticals. Accepting herbal treatments as a component of managing pneumonia is in line with the larger movement in healthcare toward integrative and customized treatment, where people look for a balance between conventional and complementary therapies.

AN OVERVIEW OF THE SYMPTOMS OF PNEUMONIA

It is essential to comprehend the general idea of pneumonia and the symptoms that are connected with it to fully recognize the importance of herbal medicines. When pus, mucus, and other inflammatory materials fill the lungs' air sacs, or alveoli, pneumonia results. This buildup can make it more difficult for the lungs to exchange carbon dioxide and oxygen, which can result in symptoms like fever, chest pain, coughing, and shortness of breath. All ages can be affected by pneumonia, but certain groups are more vulnerable to serious complications than others, including the elderly, small children, and people with compromised immune systems.

The variety of symptoms linked to pneumonia highlights how difficult it is to diagnose and cure. In traditional medicine, the specific pathogen causing the infection is targeted with the prescription of antibiotics or antiviral drugs. Herbal therapies, however, have become recognized as a potential supplemental option as the medical world struggles with problems like antibiotic resistance and the limitations of traditional treatments. Herbs with immune-stimulating qualities include licorice root, garlic, and echinacea; thyme and oregano are known for their antibacterial qualities. Incorporating these herbal treatments into management strategies for pneumonia may help improve the general health of those who suffer from this respiratory ailment in addition to treating its symptoms.

The ability of herbal medicines for pneumonia to offer a comprehensive and natural approach to treating the symptoms of this lung infection is what makes them so important. People and medical experts are looking at alternative ways to control pneumonia as awareness of the drawbacks and adverse effects of traditional therapies increases. The summary of pneumonia and its symptoms highlights the importance of a thorough and individualized treatment plan, in which herbal remedies are beneficial in fostering respiratory health and general well-being. Herbal therapies may be increasingly frequently incorporated into conventional healthcare procedures as research in this area advances, providing people with a more varied and patient-centered approach to managing pneumonia.

CHAPTER TWO

COMPREHENDING PNEUMONIA

PNEUMONIA: DEFINITION AND TYPES

A respiratory illness called pneumonia causes swelling of the air sacs in one or both lungs, which results in the accumulation of fluid or pus. Numerous microbes, including bacteria, viruses, and fungi, can be the cause of this illness. The infection causes symptoms including fever, coughing, and trouble breathing by interfering with the lungs' normal function. Pneumonia can be categorized into many categories according to the population afflicted and the agent causing the illness. Outside of hospital settings, community-acquired pneumonia (CAP) is usually caused by germs like Streptococcus pneumoniae. Methicillin-resistant Staphylococcus aureus (MRSA) is one type of drug-resistant bacteria that can cause hospital-acquired pneumonia (HAP), which is typically acquired during a hospital stay. Whereas viral pneumonia is brought on by viruses such as the respiratory syncytial virus (RSV) or influenza, aspiration pneumonia is the consequence of breathing foreign materials into the lungs.

REASONS AND DANGER ELEMENTS

Pneumonia can have many different causes, but the main ones are infectious agents. Haemophilus influenzae, Mycoplasma pneumoniae, and Streptococcus pneumoniae are frequently the causes of bacterial pneumonia. Adenoviruses, respiratory syncytial viruses (RSV), and influenza viruses are frequently linked to viral pneumonia. Though less frequent, species like Cryptococcus neoformans and Histoplasma capsulatum can cause fungal pneumonia. Additional risk factors for pneumonia include age (older people and the very young are more vulnerable), compromised immune systems, long-term conditions like diabetes or COPD, and lifestyle choices like smoking or binge drinking. Aspiring stomach or mouth contents into the lungs or breathing respiratory droplets carrying infectious organisms are the two most common ways that people get pneumonia.

CONVENTIONAL THERAPIES AND THEIR RESTRICTIONS

Antibiotics are usually prescribed for bacterial infections and antiviral drugs for viral instances of pneumonia. It's also usual practice to advise bed rest, fluids, and over-the-counter drugs to relieve symptoms. Antibiotic efficacy, however, can be restricted in viral pneumonia patients, emphasizing the significance of a precise diagnosis. Additionally, the emergence of bacterial species resistant to antibiotics presents a serious threat to established therapeutic approaches. One of the most important ways to manage pneumonia is by vaccination, as there are vaccinations against specific viruses and bacteria. Pneumonia continues to be a major global health concern despite these preventive measures, particularly among disadvantaged populations.

Antibiotic resistance is not the only limitation of pneumonia treatment. The absence of quick diagnostic tools might occasionally make it more difficult to determine the cause of an illness and recommend targeted treatments. Furthermore, especially in environments with low resources, access to healthcare resources, such as modern medical facilities and efficient treatments, might be a constraint. To address these issues, new therapeutic modalities—such as newer antibiotics and antiviral medications—must be continuously developed. To stop pneumonia from spreading and lessen its effects on global health, improved surveillance and public health initiatives are also essential. In summary, effective prevention and treatment efforts for pneumonia require a thorough understanding of the respiratory infection, including its description, forms, causes, and related risk factors.

CHAPTER THREE
OVERVIEW OF HERBAL REMEDIES
HERBAL MEDICINE'S PAST

Herbal medicine has a long history that may be traced back to the customs of many ancient societies. Herbal treatments have been an essential part of traditional medical systems for thousands of years. Similar to this, Ayurveda, the traditional medicine of India, mainly relies on the use of herbs and botanicals, as evidenced by ancient texts like the "Charaka Samhita" and "Sushruta Samhita." Herbal medicine, for example, was an integral part of traditional Chinese medicine (TCM) in ancient China, with formulations documented in texts like the "Shennong Ben Cao Jing."

Herbal medicine has a long history in the West, dating back to the times of ancient Greece and Rome. The herbal traditions of Europe have been greatly affected by the writings of famous people such as Hippocrates and Dioscorides. Monasteries developed into hubs for the production of therapeutic herbs during the Middle Ages, and generations of people retained and transmitted their knowledge of plants.

Herbalists such as John Gerard and Nicholas Culpeper contributed to the literature on herbs throughout the Renaissance, which saw a resurgence of interest in herbal medicine. Many herbal traditions came together and adapted to different cultural contexts over time, creating a wide range of herbal treatments that are used all over the world.

BENEFITS OF USING HERBAL TREATMENTS

Numerous benefits that come with using herbal medicines explain why they are still in use today and why they are so popular. Herbal medicine's holistic approach, which addresses the root causes of sickness rather than just treating its symptoms, is one of its main benefits. Herbs frequently contain a complex mixture of active ingredients that interact with one another to provide a broad range of medicinal effects.

In addition, compared to their pharmaceutical competitors, herbal medicines are often thought to be more environmentally friendly and sustainable. The increased emphasis on sustainable practices worldwide is in line with the production of medicinal plants, which frequently use fewer synthetic chemicals and have a smaller ecological impact.

The availability of herbal therapies is an additional benefit. You may grow a lot of the herbs used in traditional medicine in your backyard garden or buy them from local markets. People feel more empowered to take control of their health and well-being as a result of this accessibility.

Additionally, compared to conventional medications, herbal therapies frequently have fewer negative effects. Although there are hazards involved, the milder form of many herbal remedies can reduce negative effects when used correctly. Because of this, herbal therapy may be a desirable alternative, particularly for people who are allergic to certain pharmaceuticals or are looking for alternatives to traditional therapies.

SAFETY AND PRECAUTIONS

Herbal medicines are widely used and thought to be safe, but it's important to use caution when using them because of possible combinations and negative effects. Herbal products can differ greatly in terms of potency and purity, unlike medicines. Ensuring efficacy and safety requires quality control, and procuring herbs from reliable vendors is advised.

Some herbs have the potential to worsen pre-existing medical issues or interact with drugs. To prevent any negative reactions, people should let their healthcare practitioners know about any herbal supplements they are using. Before adding herbal treatments to their healthcare regimen, people with chronic medical illnesses, women who are pregnant, and nursing mothers should proceed with extra caution and professional assistance.

CHAPTER FOUR

MEDICINAL COMPONENTS FOR PNEUMONIA

EUCALYPTUS

A popular herbal treatment with a long history of use, eucalyptus relieves the symptoms of respiratory disorders, including pneumonia. The eucalyptus tree produces anti-inflammatory and antibacterial chemicals in its leaves, such as eucalyptol. These qualities have the potential to lessen respiratory tract irritation and fight infections that could lead to pneumonia. Furthermore, it's thought that breathing in eucalyptus oil vapors would relax the respiratory system and lessen breathing problems.

THYME

Another herb with a long history of medical usage is thyme, which has antibacterial and anti-inflammatory qualities due to its constituents like thymol. Thyme has been used historically to improve respiratory health; its expectorant properties may help to facilitate mucus release and facilitate easier expulsion. This can be especially helpful in cases of pneumonia, as the buildup of mucus in the lungs can make breathing more difficult.

OREGANO

Compounds with antibacterial and anti-inflammatory activities, such as carvacrol and rosmarinic acid, are found in oregano, a culinary herb with noteworthy therapeutic benefits. The plant's leaves are used to make oregano oil, which has been studied for its ability to treat respiratory infections. Because of its antibacterial qualities, the body's natural defenses against pneumonia may be strengthened by preventing the growth of germs in the lungs.

GARLIC

Due to its immune-stimulating qualities, garlic has long been used to treat a variety of respiratory ailments. One of the main ingredients in garlic, allicin, is known to have antibacterial properties. Garlic may be able to lessen the symptoms of respiratory distress and assist fight against pathogenic organisms that cause pneumonia.

GINGER

Due to its well-known anti-inflammatory and antioxidant qualities, ginger has been used as a treatment for respiratory conditions. The main ingredient in ginger, gingerol, has the potential to lessen respiratory tract inflammation and lessen the signs and symptoms of respiratory infections. Furthermore, ginger's warming qualities are supposed to encourage circulation, which may strengthen the immune system.

ROOT LICORICE

Because licorice root helps relieve respiratory irritation, it has been utilized in traditional medicine. Glycyrrhizin, one of the licorice's constituents, has anti-inflammatory qualities. This herbal remedy has the potential to alleviate airway irritation and alleviate pneumonia symptoms. It's crucial to remember that licorice overconsumption should be avoided owing to possible negative effects.

MULLEIN

Mullein has long been used to treat respiratory problems because of its expectorant qualities. Saponins found in mullein plant leaves may aid in loosening mucus and facilitate its removal from the respiratory system. In cases of pneumonia, where efficient mucus clearance is essential for respiratory function, this can be especially helpful.

SAGE

The potential of sage, a fragrant herb with antibacterial properties, to treat respiratory infections has been investigated. Thujone and camphor are two of the chemicals in sage that may be involved in its antibacterial properties. During pneumonia, sage tea or sage vapor inhalation may be beneficial for respiratory health.

ANDROGRAPHIS

Native to South Asian nations, Andrographis is a plant whose possible immune-stimulating qualities have drawn interest. Andrographolides, the active ingredients, have antiviral and anti-inflammatory properties. Although there is little study on Andrographis about pneumonia, the plant's historical use for respiratory ailments raises the possibility of immune system support advantages.

It is best to work with a healthcare provider to integrate these herbal substances into a comprehensive therapy plan for pneumonia. Although these herbs have shown potential in traditional medicine, there is still a growing body of scientific evidence to support their efficacy in treating pneumonia. It's critical to speak with a healthcare professional to decide whether to combine traditional medical treatments with herbal therapies safely and appropriately.

CHAPTER FIVE

ADMINISTRATION AND PREPARATION
TEAS AND INFUSIONS

Herbal remedies and plant-based compounds are often prepared and consumed as infusions and teas. Herbs or plant materials are steeped in boiling water to extract their therapeutic properties, a process known as infusion. For sensitive plant parts like leaves and flowers, which can be harmed by more forceful extraction techniques, this procedure is frequently utilized.

To make an infusion, the plant material is usually covered with boiling water and steeped for a predetermined amount of time. In essence, teas are infusions, however, the terms are occasionally used synonymously. These preparations are valued for their healing properties as well as the ritualistic comfort that comes with making and eating them.

TINCTURES

Another method of preparing herbs is the creation of tinctures, which are made by extracting therapeutic components with alcohol or a water-and-alcohol mixture. This technique works especially well for extracting a variety of components, such as molecules that are soluble in alcohol and water. Herbal treatments can be administered more concentratedly and conveniently using tinctures since the liquid form makes dosage management easier.

The alcohol component prolongs the tincture's shelf life by acting as a preservative. The proportion of alcohol and the length of the extraction process can change depending on the plant and its characteristics, which can affect the tincture's potency and efficacy.

APPLY POULTICES

Herbal materials are applied externally to the skin directly as poultices. Applying a soft, wet mass of ground or crushed herbs often combined with water or another liquid to the affected area is the goal of this treatment. Poultices have several uses, such as reducing swelling, encouraging the healing of wounds, and pulling out toxins. The poultice's warmth promotes blood circulation in the targeted area, which furthers the therapeutic effects, and the direct touch with the skin facilitates the absorption of advantageous substances.

BREATHS

Herbal medications are inhaled and administered through the respiratory system. When it comes to treating respiratory conditions like sinusitis, congestion, and coughing, this strategy works very well. A popular method is steam inhalation, which involves breathing in hot water infused with herbs to allow the healing vapors to enter the respiratory system.

In this mode of administration, volatile plant materials such as essential oils, herbs, or other plant components are frequently utilized. These volatile substances can directly affect the respiratory system by inhalation, relieving symptoms, and enhancing respiratory health.

GUIDELINES FOR DOSAGE

The safe and efficient use of herbal remedies depends on following dosage recommendations. The right dosage is determined by several variables, including the user's weight, age, health, and the particular herb or treatment being used. It is imperative to adhere to dosage recommendations made by medical professionals, herbalists, or other reliable sources. Certain herbs might have negative consequences if used in excess, which emphasizes the need for responsible and knowledgeable use. Furthermore, since each person's reaction to herbal medicines may be different, it's best to begin with smaller doses and raise them gradually as needed, keeping an eye out for any negative side effects.

A variety of techniques are used in the preparation and administration of herbal remedies, all of which are designed to extract and deliver the therapeutic components of plants. Teas and infusions, tinctures, poultices, and inhalations provide unique methods to address a range of health issues. To ensure the safe and efficient use of these herbal remedies and support a holistic approach to well-being, it is essential to understand the appropriate dosage parameters.

HERBAL MIXTURES OPTIMAL MIXTURES FOR PNEUMONIA

When it comes to herbal remedies, the idea of synergistic combinations is especially important when treating ailments like pneumonia. Because pneumonia is characterized by inflammation of the lung tissue, treating the condition holistically can help reduce symptoms and accelerate healing. To create a more potent and efficient treatment, synergistic blends strategically combine different herbs to boost each other's therapeutic capabilities.

Herbs having expectorant, antibacterial, and anti-inflammatory qualities are frequently used in conjunction to have a synergistic effect for treating pneumonia. For instance, combining thyme, which has antibacterial characteristics, with herbs like Echinacea, which is recognized for immune-boosting capabilities, can result in a potent combination to fight the pathogenic organisms that cause pneumonia. This combination helps the body's immunological response while also addressing the underlying problem.

MAKING CUSTOMIZED HERBAL COMBINATIONS

A customized approach to herbal treatment is represented by personalized herbal formulae, which acknowledge that people may react differently to different herbs depending on their constitution, medical history, and particular symptoms. This method entails a comprehensive evaluation of a person's physical, mental, and lifestyle aspects to craft a custom herbal formula that meets their unique requirements.

A customized herbal recipe for pneumonia may include the patient's immune system strength, the intensity of their symptoms, and any underlying medical issues. For example, someone with a history of respiratory problems can find relief from inflamed airways with herbs like licorice and mullein, while someone with a compromised immune system could need extra immune-stimulating herbs like astragalus.

COMPLEMENTARY HERBS

By offering extra support or reducing possible adverse effects, complementary herbs are essential for optimizing the overall efficacy of a herbal solution. Complementary herbs are selected to function in conjunction with the main herbs in the formula to cure pneumonia by addressing secondary symptoms, enhancing general well-being, or preventing any possible negative effects.

For example, although the main herbs for treating pneumonia are garlic and oregano, you can also include complementing herbs, such as marshmallow root or slippery elm, to help soothe inflamed mucous membranes and reduce coughing. This well-rounded strategy guarantees a more thorough and well-rounded treatment in addition to addressing the main issue.

Complementary herbs, individualized herbal formulations, and synergistic blends are essential to using herbal medicine to treat pneumonia effectively. Through an understanding of the distinct qualities of many herbs and how they interact, both individuals and herbalists can develop individualized, comprehensive strategies to promote respiratory health and general well-being.

CHAPTER SIX

COMBINING CONVENTIONAL MEDICINE WITH HERBAL REMEDIES

WORKING TOGETHER WITH MEDICAL PROFESSIONALS

When combining herbal therapies with traditional medicine, patients and medical professionals must work together to find alternate solutions. To guarantee a thorough grasp of the patient's health profile, it is imperative to establish open communication and transparency between patients and their healthcare providers.

Within this cooperative framework, medical practitioners are essential in assessing the efficacy and safety of herbal treatments, taking into account any possible drug interactions, and resolving any negative effects concerns. This collaboration creates an atmosphere in which patients are more equipped to decide whether to use herbal treatments in their entire healthcare regimen.

POSSIBLE ADVANTAGES AND HAZARDS

Combining herbal medicines with traditional medicine has several possible advantages as well as disadvantages. Herbal remedies, which are frequently made from plants and other natural sources, may have medicinal qualities that enhance traditional medical care. Relieving symptoms, enhancing well-being, and assisting the body's natural healing processes are a few possible advantages.

But it's important to be aware of the possible risks that come with using herbal therapies, like inconsistent dosage, inconsistent product quality, and a lack of established guidelines. Moreover, there is a chance that some herbal supplements will negatively interact with prescription medications, reducing their effectiveness or resulting in unexpected side effects. To guarantee the security and efficacy of integrated healthcare systems, a comprehensive evaluation of these advantages and hazards is required.

DEVELOPING A BALANCED STRATEGY

A comprehensive grasp of each person's unique health requirements and preferences is necessary to develop a balanced strategy for combining herbal medicines with conventional medication. Patients should work to achieve a harmonious balance between evidence-based conventional therapy and herbal remedies, in cooperation with healthcare specialists. This entails taking into account the seriousness of the ailment, the reliability of the scientific data about herbal treatments, and the possibility of cooperative treatment programs. A balanced strategy promotes a comprehensive view of healthcare that acknowledges the importance of both conventional and cutting-edge therapeutic techniques. It also emphasizes how crucial it is to continuously monitor and reevaluate the integrated treatment plan to modify it in response to the patient's response and any new medical advancements.

The fusion of traditional medicine and herbal medicines is a complicated but growingly common facet of modern medicine. To properly navigate this integration, ensure informed decision-making, and minimize potential hazards, collaboration with healthcare experts is essential. Both patients and healthcare professionals must be aware of the possible advantages and disadvantages of using herbal treatments. In the end, achieving a balanced strategy necessitates a careful and customized evaluation of the patient's health, integrating the benefits of both conventional and herbal techniques to maximize general well-being.

CHAPTER SEVEN

DIETARY AND LIFESTYLE SUGGESTIONS

NUTRITION AS A TOOL FOR RECOVERY SUPPORT

Whether the body is recovering from an illness, accident, or other health issue, nutrition is essential to its healing process. A diet rich in nutrients and well-balanced is crucial for giving the body the building blocks it needs to heal wounds, strengthen the immune system, and reestablish general health. Eating a diet high in vitamins, minerals, and antioxidants is crucial during recovery since these nutrients help to reduce inflammation and promote healing.

The mainstay of a diet centered on recovery should be protein, as it is essential for tissue regeneration. Essential amino acids are found in foods like lean meats, fish, eggs, dairy products, and plant-based foods like tofu and lentils. These amino acids aid in the body's healing processes.

A varied spectrum of vitamins and antioxidants is ensured by including a choice of vibrant fruits and vegetables, bolstering the immune system and thwarting oxidative damage.

Another essential component of diet during recovery is hydration. Maintaining adequate hydration is essential for effective healing since it facilitates the removal of toxins, enhances organ function, and preserves cellular hydration. Drinking enough water, herbal teas, and electrolyte-rich liquids can all make a big difference in the healing process.

MODIFICATIONS TO LIFESTYLE FOR RESPIRATORY HEALTH

Overall well-being depends on having a healthy respiratory system, and making specific lifestyle adjustments can improve lung function and respiratory capacity. Keeping the atmosphere smoke-free is essential since both tobacco smoke and other environmental toxins can seriously harm respiratory health.

Reducing time spent in places with poor air quality and avoiding secondhand smoke exposure can help prevent respiratory problems and enhance lung health.

Apart from environmental factors, it is imperative to include consistent physical exercise in one's routine to maintain respiratory health. Exercise increases lung capacity, strengthens respiratory muscles, and improves cardiovascular fitness in general. Exercises like cycling, swimming, jogging, and brisk walking can help to keep respiratory function at its best.

Additionally, engaging in mindfulness activities and deep breathing exercises might help to relax the respiratory muscles and expand the lungs. For people with respiratory disorders, breathing exercises like diaphragmatic and pursed-lip breathing can be very helpful as they enhance oxygen exchange and reduce symptoms like dyspnea.

EXERCISE AND METHODS FOR BREATHING

Exercise is crucial for maintaining respiratory health in addition to its importance for general physical health. Running, cycling, and other aerobic exercises are examples of cardiovascular exercises that increase lung capacity and oxygen exchange efficiency. Regular exercise also helps you stay at a healthy weight, which eases the burden on your respiratory system.

Certain breathing exercises can improve respiratory function even more than general exercise. A deep inhalation is required for diaphragmatic breathing, also known as belly breathing, which causes the lungs to fill with air and the diaphragm to descend. This method can help manage stress and anxiety, which can hurt respiratory health, while also promoting effective oxygen exchange.

Another method is pursed-lip breathing, which is breathing in through the nose and out through the lips. This aids in lowering the rate of breathing, preventing airway collapse, and enhancing the expulsion of stagnant air from the lungs. These breathing exercises are especially beneficial for people who have respiratory diseases including chronic obstructive pulmonary disease (COPD) or asthma. Maintaining good respiratory health can be greatly aided by incorporating targeted breathing exercises and exercise into one's routine.

CHAPTER EIGHT

HERBAL TREATMENTS FOR AVOIDANCE

BOOST IMMUNE SYSTEM POWER

Herbal medicine is a comprehensive method that has been used for ages in many different cultures to strengthen the immune system. The immune system is essential for protecting the body from diseases and infections. The immune-stimulating qualities of herbs like echinacea, astragalus, and elderberry are widely documented. For example, astragalus has long been used in Chinese medicine to promote immune function generally, and echinacea is thought to increase immune cell activity. If one incorporates these herbs into their regular regimen, it can help maintain a strong immune system.

DEVELOPING RESPIRATORY HARDINESS

Herbal medicines for prevention also play a significant role in strengthening respiratory resilience. Because the respiratory system is susceptible to environmental influences and viruses, strengthening its defenses is crucial. Herbs that are well known for their respiratory benefits include licorice root, thyme, and oregano. Compounds with antibacterial qualities found in oregano and thyme help to prevent respiratory infections. Conversely, licorice root is well-known for its calming effects on the respiratory system, which support good respiratory health in general. Making tinctures or teas with these herbs can be a useful strategy to enhance respiratory resistance.

LONG-TERM HEALTH STRATEGIES

Herbal medicines are an essential component of long-term health initiatives since they promote overall well-being. Herbs that are known to assist the body in adapting to stimuli and maintaining equilibrium include ashwagandha and holy basil. These herbs support long-term vitality in addition to addressing current health issues. Furthermore, adding antioxidant-rich plants to the diet, such as ginger and turmeric, can reduce inflammation and oxidative stress while enhancing general health and longevity.

POSSIBILITIES AND DIFFICULTIES

A sophisticated awareness of each person's unique health demands is necessary to successfully navigate the potential and difficulties offered by herbal therapies for prevention. Herbal medicines provide a natural and frequently kinder approach to health, but it's important to take into account things like personal sensitivities and possible drug combinations. A skilled healthcare expert or herbalist can offer tailored advice, ensuring that herbal interventions support a person's desired health outcomes. Finding the ideal ratio and mix of herbs might be difficult, but with the correct support, herbal treatments can provide a long-lasting and comprehensive approach to preventive health.

Herbal medicines for prevention cover a wide range of techniques meant to fortify the immune system, develop respiratory resilience, and promote long-term health practices. To fully embrace the benefits of nature's pharmacopeia, one must be aware of the many uses of herbs and how they may enhance general health. A thoughtful and knowledgeable approach can assist people in managing obstacles and maximizing the preventative health benefits that herbal treatments can offer when they begin their herbal journey.